Sheik Nazim al

Natural Medicin

Natural Medicines

traditional sufi healing methods

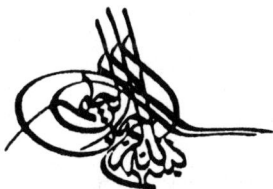

Sheik Nazim al Haqqani
an-Naqshbandia

ZERO PRODUCTIONS

© Thyra Quensel
August 1995

1. edition - 1989 -
2. edition -1992 -
3. edition - 1995 -

Published by: Zero Productions, London
collected, edited, commented, typeset
& illustrated by Zero

British Library Cataloguing in Publication Data.
A catalogue record for this book is availble from the British
Library

ISBN 1-898863-10-5

Printed and bound in Great Britain by
Redwood Books Ltd, Trowbridge, Wiltshire

INTRODUCTION

Maulana SHEIK NAZIM al Haqqani is the 40th Sheik in the Golden Chain of the Naqshbandi Tariqat, which leads back to the Prophet Muhammad* as the first recipient of Divine Knowledge within this line of succession.

When I first met him 13 years ago, I was dazzled by the spiritual light radiating from him. In those days he had been coming to Great Britain since 1974 to spend the Holy Month of Ramadan. This was one of the last orders he received from his Master Sheik Abdullah Daghistani. He had been told, that the Last Days were coming nearer and that the prophecy of 'the Light arising from the West' was becoming a reality.

The deep darkness reigning over the West, especially within the raw jungle of overcivilized cities, is a result of disbelief and unwillingness to follow Divine Orders, which have been sent down regularly to mankind since Adam. 'We shall be like stars in the sky!' proclaimed the Prophet Muhammad*.

One day a young lady came to Sheik Nazim, who had been diagnosed as having cancer in her thyroid. The doctors wanted to start operating, but she did not want any knife to cut into her throat. Sheik Nazim told her to start drinking onion-juice every morning before

---

* May peace be upon him.

taking anything else. After repeating the 40-day treatment, she was completely cured. This was partly very embarrassing, because she had applied for a pension and the doctors could not find a trace of the cancer anymore!

From that day on I started collecting the medical advice which Sheik Nazim was giving to ill people who had asked for help. I had seen how it had been possible to cure cancer. I knew that the remedies he recommended worked. Some people were surprised and said, "But he is a spiritual teacher, not a healer." It does take quite some time to even begin to understand the endless horizons of what the Man of Time, the Saint of Saints can do.

Zero Quensel

FOREWORD

In our days people are more than ever in need of new forms of medicine. Illnesses are increasing every day and it is becoming more and more impossible for physicians to find treatments, medicines or even names to cure these illnesses. With this booklet I am addressing all of mankind. I am warning all of them so they may heed to Heavenly Warnings. Everything said here has this condition. I hope it will be useful for mankind and that the Lord of Heavens may bless us endlessly so we may believe and be His good servants.

Sheik Nazim al Haqqani an Naqshbandia

WITHOUT CHEMISTRY OR KNIVES: THE PROPHETS' ART OF HEALING

Ours is the most terrible and most dangerous time for living people, because it is becoming increasingly difficult to find the right protection and cure for ever more appearing new illnesses. As long as physicians and researchers continue their studies, they will find more illnesses and develop more medicines and treatments against them. It will be impossible to make a limit. The number of illnesses and treatments existing in our days have reached a climax. At the same time it makes physicians tired and they are starting to reach a point of hopelessness. They are realising that it is impossible to try to control them or to stop their spreading.

So we are looking for some main medicine to treat mankind. We believe that illnesses, like everything else, come to the servants of the Creator through His Will. Without His Will illnesses would never come and never go. Do you think that there is another reason?

Nowadays so many medicines are being used for curing. Don't believe that these medicines and operations are of any use! If people were obedient servants, Allah Almighty would be able to give health and take away the illness. As long as people think that only medicines will take away illnesses, the illnesses will never go away.

People think that they will be cured by different pills, syrups, injections or laser-treatments. It is easy to get this impression. But the fact is, that these methods go against our natural being. Allah Almighty has created treatments for us which are natural. Chemicals destroy our bodies like poisons, because they are not of the same substance. This also applies to all kinds of radiation-treatment which hits the body like fire and burns. When one side has been burnt, the damage will spread to the whole body.

Don't think that treatment has to be artificial and that you will find cure through chemicals. The heavy pressure which artificial medicines cause, make humans tired and even lead to them losing their consciousness. Then, when the effect of the medicine and its strong poison decreases, the microbes and bacteria become even more alive and will plunge onto the organs. Allah Almighty will give them the order; "Destroy!"

The reason for all this is disobedience. People never want to consider that health is from the Creator. They think it is a result of pills and operations. That is a great sin. Some people come to me after they have asked many doctors for advice. They tell me that no-one can heal their illness. Every day new illnesses appear which cannot even be explained by professors. Partly very strange illnesses concerning eyes, ears, tongue, brain, neck, heart, liver, lungs, stomach, kidneys, bones, blood, nose...

In our days such a complexity afflicts our bodies. People get ill, feel ill, go to physicians, to laboratories, make x-rays, feel ill, go again... and after having made a full check-up the doctors tell them:

-There is nothing wrong.

-But I am ill.

-Everything is all right.

-But I feel ill.

That is another kind of punishment, to feel ill. There is no medicine, but they will get drugs to forget and cause some parts of the brain not to function. The physician will feel obliged to give drugs. Like this, even though the patient is not ill, the doctor will poison him. This is happening to millions of people.

The last thing will be that the doctors say, "We must cut your head." Then they touch the brain. This is the most difficult operation, no-one should accept it. With heart operations it is the same; it is hopeless and dangerous.

To use a knife is always harmful, but nowadays physicians mostly hurry up and cut. It is so difficult and harmful. There is a treatment for every illness without using a knife, a natural medicine. It may take more time, but it has no side effects.

Nearly every treatment ends in an operation, and operations are no real cures. It is only in this century that doctors have started to use operations in such an exaggerated way. Today they are the main element in treatment of illnesses. Nearly every doctor seems to have nothing else in mind than to cut. They want to cut, sew, add something and destroy, nothing else. That is not a treatment, it is a punishment!

Illness is a punishment for people living in our days. Only a small percentage of the people have not had a knife cutting their body. That is one way in which this punishment reaches the whole world from East to West. After getting the punishment, the form of treatment they ask for is the next punishment. The result is that they can become crippled. In our days every part of the body has been cut and opened and has suffered: the head, heart, liver... All this is another punishment. It will not give the patient rest, never! It is not a treatment.

People of the 20th century have lost their patience. Mankind has no more patience. They want quick treatment. The cures through natural medicines take time, but mankind has no patience and want their pain and suffering to stop quickly. That is why they are willing to take strong new artificial medicines. It doesn't matter to them if these harm their bodies. Their only interest is to stop the pain and suffering quickly.

And so, the more patient a patient can be, and the more natural medicine they use, the better. Operations should be avoided, because to cut into our body does not suit our nature. Our body is like a closed box. If someone opens it and then tries to close it, it could be impossible. Even experts might have difficulties in putting it back the way it was again. This can even happen to famous surgeons. Because every body is different and it could be difficult to find out what should be removed. Or maybe something remains which should have been taken out. It is like when you try to pull out the roots of a tree; you might leave a piece inside which you didn't see. You will celebrate that the big piece is out, and then, a year later, the small piece which was left behind will have grow and become big. That is another reason why operations are so dangerous. We must try never to touch our bodies in such a way.

We must try to use natural medicines, cures which our Creator has created for us. The more patient a patient is, and the more he relies on the power of natural medicines, the better. These are the same medicines which have been used since thousands of years, since beginning of time. Usually the knowledge of such medicines have come to us through Heavenly Beings, Prophets or Messengers. The wisdom of such teachings have been concluded through the Divine Art of Healing of our beloved Seal of Prophets, Muhammad, may peace be with him. It is important to listen to him, because Allah Almighty has given him Heavenly Knowledge which includes the cure for every illness.

We advise you to use Divine Methods of Treatment. They consist in simple natural medicines. Our bodies belong to nature, so the cure can only come from nature. All artificial methods which are so common nowadays, go against the nature of mankind. That is why it has to stop. Every artificial, synthetic medicine attacks the natural substance of our body. We must prevent that, because it causes great harm.

So be patient, as patient as can be. If someone isn't patient, he must seek a cure as quickly as possible. If he doesn't know any natural medicine, then he has to take another one. But natural medicines made out of herbs and plants will always be the best. Slowly, very slowly Europeans and Western societies are coming back to the wisdom of using natural medicines.

THERE IS A CURE FOR EVERY ILLNESS

Simple illnesses have simple medicines. But during the development of mankind and the increase of disobedience, the illnesses have also started to be disobedient towards medicines and cannot be cured anymore. By the permission of Allah Almighty a very grave illness can also be defeated by a simple medicine, but the more mankind has become disloyal and disobedient to Divine Laws, the more illnesses have become impossible to cure, even the most simple ones.

Our Grandsheik[1] always used to say, "If someone has the dangerous illness cancer, they should drink onion juice. That is the best." Sometimes people say that they have already tried hundreds of different medicines and still the terrible illness will not go away. But if they start to drink onion juice, it will.

The Prophet Abraham* said, "When I am ill, Allah will take the illness from me and make me healthy again." Some people are on the level, that when they

---

1 Grandsheik Abdullah Faiz Daghistani is the teacher of Sheik Nazim and his predecessor in the Golden Chain of the Order of the Naqshbandia.

are ill they do not need medicine. That is then all right. For example, when Abu Bakr* was ill, the people wanted to bring a doctor to him. But he said, "The doctor will make me ill. From where is the doctor coming?" What he meant, was that Allah was going to cure him. Everything comes from Him, and so he thought it unnecessary that anyone else should try to take it away, because only Allah can do that.

With Moses* it was a completely different story: he had a headache, a very strong headache. The Children of Israel sent their doctors to him and said, "Use this!". "No!" was his reply. Someone else came and brought him another medicine and asked him to use it. Again he refused. Then Allah Almighty sent the Angel Gabriel to Moses to order him to use a medicine., "Oh Moses, I have created so many cures in the different plants and herbs so that my people may find the cure in them. So much in this world is a cure. All of this I created for mankind, so that they may use it. Do you want to make the wisdom I put into it worthless? Is it your wish to become healthy again without using this? If you do not, I will not give you back your health. Because if I would, the wisdom which I put into creating them, would be of no importance anymore."

This is as an example for mankind in general. That is why Allah Almighty commanded him to use medicine to get well. You should also use it. At the same time, if I would recite on water and give it to you as a medicine, then you might say that it was the water that cured you. That would be silly. It is not the water that will give you your health back, it is Allah who gives it through the water.

I say to you, "Use onion juice and it will give you health, *insha'Allah*." Don't say, "I am using 100 different medicines and nothing can stop it, so how can you say that the onion juice will? " I am not saying that it is the onion juice that will stop the illness, but that which Allah Almighty has put in it as a cure.

Once I visited a doctor in Karachi, Pakistan. It was a simple clinic. A Holy Verse from the Holy Quran was written over the door, 'And when I am ill, it is He Who cures me.' (26:80). This is a great warning and over the door it drew the attention of everyone coming to that doctor. It would not be correct to blame it on the doctor if someone does not get cured. The cure does not come from the doctor and from the medicines, but from Allah. When people left this belief and left paradise, thousands and thousands of illnesses befell them, even though there are only 360 organs in the body.

We believe that there are many reasons for people to become ill. Some are physical, some are spiritual. As believers we do not accept that every illness only comes from a disease and only has something to do with physical life. There is also a Heavenly Reaction which affects people and makes them ill.

CHARITIES

All Prophets advised their nations, their believers and their followers to use charity as a protection against illnesses. This is not only an Islamic wisdom. Every religion has declared the importance of giving or doing an act of charity. Before even trying any medicine, people must try to cure themselves through charity.

When this has been understood, treatment is easy for believers. For unbelievers the cure is very difficult. The soul helps the believer to be cured, but the souls of unbelievers are against them and will never support them. So the cure of unbelievers takes longer and longer and might even stay until the last moment of their lives. Believers, on the other hand, because their souls support them, can quickly be treated and cured.

So the most important foundation for the treatment and cure of illnesses, is to give charity.

THE ART OF PREVENTIVE MEDICINE

The most important condition for any cure or prevention of illness, is the belief in one God, in His Unity and that everything comes through His Will. Some illnesses come as a punishment for disobedience and some come as a test for His servants to see, if they accept it. He sends goodness and badness, poverty and wealth, illness and health. He gives honour and He humiliates. He gives power and He gives weakness, difficulties and ease.

Being the Lord of mankind, He has the right to test them and to tempt them, to see if they remain true to Him and to His way, or if they sway and turn away, or if they remain obedient and remain His servants in all situations.

This is the belief in *Qadr*, the belief that we are under Divine Destiny and Arrangement, that every thing which happens, happens through the Will of Allah. The wisdom which lies behind this, is the test for His servants, to see if they are obedient and respectful to Him always, under all conditions.

That is why we are saying that everyone must believe in the existence of the Lord of the Heavens, must believe in the Creator of the whole universe and must believe in His Will and Power. They must also believe that the treatment of His servants can only come about by His Will. Only if He wills it, can treatment come to the people, to ill people. If He does not want it, only more punishment will come, not treatment.

With my given authority I am advising all of mankind to hear and to listen to the words of the Lord. If they are not listening and obeying, punishment will just come on them every day and there will be no treatment and no cure for them. There will be no happiness and no rest for their bodies or minds or hearts.

This means to listen to the Messengers of the Lord, including the last one, Sayyidina Muhammad*. Allah Almighty taught him every kind of treatment. Every illness is well known to the Seal of Prophets and he has been given Heavenly Knowledge concerning the medicines and treatments for all of them.

Mankind must try to keep their bodies safe. The way of doing this, is to keep everything away which harms the body. All of this is mentioned in the Heavenly Messages. You must try to keep these rules and stay away from everything which damages and harms. Everything which harms is mentioned in the Holy Books and is prohibited by the Lord Almighty Allah. As long as you go against these rules, you will be punished and find no treatment.

Illnesses never come without a reason: either it is as a punishment to make the person obey, or it is to demonstrate the treatment for others. Whoever drinks alcohol must be punished. All drinks that harm the body are prohibited and should not be drunk. Anyone who opposes this and says, "Oh, just a little bit..." will be punished just a little bit. If a person takes a little bit of poison, he will suffer a little bit. If he takes more, he will suffer more. This is because prohibited things are poison, spiritually and physically.

If anyone smokes, he must be punished. If he only smokes a little bit, then he must also only be punished a little bit. If very much, the punishment will be very big. If anyone eats pork and that which is prohibited of dead animals, it will harm the body and there will come a punishment. If a man and a woman do illegal acts: once twice or three times, something can attack her and him and they will be punished. Until people leave all these things which I am mentioning, they will be punished sooner or later.

In the West people are usually not careful with what they eat. They do not vary their diet. They stick to hamburgers, Kentucky Fried Chicken and Indian food. But Allah Almighty created so many kinds of foods. Fruits, for example, prevent infections in the organs. Instead people drink so much artificial things which cause infections. Allah Almighty created 4 seasons with different foods. People are supposed to eat the fruits and the vegetables of the season because they contain the substances needed for those weather conditions. People in Cyprus are still accustomed to eat fresh tomatoes, aubergines, okra, cucumbers, melons... But here in the West, because of all the hormones and imports, you can get all kinds at all times. In the old days people would look forward to the fruit of the season.

At the time of the Prophet Muhammad* most of the people were ignorant of any Heavenly Rules and they were doing everything they wanted. Then Islam came, they accepted it and were purified by following the Lord's Command. If anyone today is acting wrong out of ignorance and then submits and says, "Oh, my Lord, I will not do these things again, I am listening and obeying You!" then the illness can be removed through Divine Will without using any medicine, even illnesses like Aids. When disbelief, *Kufr*, is taken away, everything else that is bad is taken away too. But it must be realised that every prohibited action brings illnesses, unknown illnesses. In our days unknown illnesses are coming to us through homosexual people and there is no treatment and no medicine for them because they are going against the Holy Command of the Lord of Heavens. If they find a cure another hopeless illness will come, because the Creator can create so many bacteria and viruses. It is endless...

So the first protection is not to put the body in front of danger. In the same way as someone who puts their hand on an electric wire will feel the painful result.

The parents of children born with diseases are the ones being punished, not the children. If people take care, then they are protected. For such people it is easy to be treated. Even water, the source of life, gives them treatment and can be a medicine.

Allah created cold and hot water. You may lie in cold water or in hot water or in mud and your body can be renewed. You may drink some water and it can clean your inside. You may eat grapes and it will be like a medicine. You may eat melon and it will give you strength. You may eat wheat and it will give you power. Everything which we are using as a grace or as a favour from Allah Almighty will at the same time be a source of power and a medicine for us. In that way here is no need to look for other medicines because the Lord of Heavens, the Lord of the children of Adam, created everything and gave a treatment for everything. Life power is in every food and likewise every food is a medicine. The only condition is to start every meal by praising and thanking Him, "In the name of Allah Who created this for His servants' wealth and health!" every time before eating or drinking. Use everything in His Name, and it will be a treatment and medicine for you.

That is the only purpose for which the Lord created it, not to be avoided. Nowadays when you go to famous physicians they will list up endlessly which foods you are to avoid, "Don't eat this, don't touch that, don't use that..." This is not a treatment but a punishment. It is because you were using all that nourishment without mentioning the Lord, without being grateful to Him. So He takes it away from you! For some people it is never-ending, "Don't eat sugar, don't eat fruits, don't eat meat, don't touch butter, don't touch honey..."

It is also very important to follow the *sunna*, the traditions of the prophets, especially of the last one, Sayyidina Muhammad*, because his have been most accurately recorded.

In those days Muhammad* sent a letter to the King of Egypt who was very grateful and sent back a present. It was a donkey, a servant and a doctor. Muhammad accepted it and said, "We can use the servant as a helper because we have so many guests every day. The donkey is also very useful to help us carry our heavy loads. But we don't need a doctor." But the doctor insisted that he had been ordered to serve him, and so the Prophet told him that he could stay as long as he wanted.

The doctor stayed for one year, and then asked for permission to leave. The Prophet asked why, and the doctor replied that during one year not one single person had come to complain about any kind of illness, not even a headache, toothache or a stomach-ache.

Muhammad* said, "We are never ill, because we never eat until we are hungry and we don't eat too much, we always leave a small part empty."

"Yes," said the doctor, "like that no illness will ever come to you."

On another occasion the Prophet said that we should leave 1/3 for food, 1/3 for drink and 1/3 for air in the stomach. Nowadays people eat until they are full. Even then they want more. Like cows and oxen they eat without a break; sweets and chocolates non-stop. This is a typical characteristic of animals: to be busy with their physical bodies all the time by eating, drinking, smoking... until it is time to go to sleep. They never give their stomach a break. And so, if one of the main reasons for illnesses is a too full stomach, then of course fasting is a main cure.

Eat only two meals a day. When you keep your stomach busy, the body is weakened because when your stomach is full, the blood is busy with digestion and has no time to fight the bacteria. So when you feel hungry, try to wait another one or two hours. In this time the blood can circulate and when it meets a bacteria, destroy it. The blood acts as a control organ in your body. If you keep it that way, the bacteria will stay weak and not cause any damage. The biggest wisdom is to remain hungry if you want to be healthy. Every illness comes to you after eating. But nowadays you will not find people who are hungry in the Western world. Everybody has to eat or drink something all the time. They even need special drinking water! They are like animals. They are nearly sleeping, and still eating nuts and chocolate. And they have hardly woken up and they already ask for their breakfast. As soon as they open their eyes they start looking for it. They never ever want to be hungry. The 20th century civilisation lets their people eat and drink too much. This puts them on the level of animals. But we have a different structure. Animals use that which they eat in a different way. The grass and the plants turn into milk, butter and wool. They eat and serve mankind with that which it becomes. But the human body does not serve anyone. For animals it is not dangerous to eat endlessly, it is part of their nature, not so for mankind.

So by eating and drinking less you will become healthier. The first thing you have to do, is to say to yourself to eat and drink less. This is why doctors prescribe diets, to enable the blood to patrol the body and combat the bacteria.

Finally people must watch the quality of what they eat. Today it is difficult to find anything which doesn't have hormones in it. From the outside it looks good, but it is full of hormones. The reason why so many hormones are being used, is that people waste about 90% of their natural resources, and so, to be able to satisfy the ever-growing needs and desires of mankind, the natural fertilizers are not enough anymore. This big waste is the reason for half of all illnesses. If mankind could change that, the illnesses would decrease quickly. Therefore it is good to buy from health-food shops. The food there is without hormones and the higher prices stop people from wasting it.

As a result of ever-growing technology, the process of preparing our natural substances have also become more and more complicated and refined. For example, when salt is refined, so many things are taken away which give benefit to the body and which the body needs. The same with olive oil: when it is refined, its natural originality changes. Everything which is refined harms mankind. They are always trying to change the natural being. They think that the Lord Almighty Allah doesn't know what is suitable for our beings, so they try to change it and to make it more suitable. That is impossible! Allah knows! For thousands of years no-one ever thought of refining olive oil. Now they remove the rich parts and use them for something else. They do not throw them away, they use them for other purposes, maybe for other oils, or margarine. They leave the olive oil without essence, and the essence is the important point in it which gives the benefit to our bodies.

They are trying everything in their minds to change as much as possible. But the best for mankind is that which Allah Almighty has created. It should be used without putting your hand to change its identity. Keep it as it is. If man eats that which comes from nature, the way it is, it is the best medicine for the physical bodies. But mankind is so involved with everything that they plant vegetables, corns and fruits and make people more sick.

So when treating illnesses with natural medicines it is first of all important to be patient. Then, when you eat, eat just a little. Don't waste anything and eat natural food from health-food shops. When preparing food, do so with a good intention. Eat with your right hand. It is *sunna* from the Prophet. Shaitan eats with his left hand. Whoever eats with the left hand damages the body.

Cleanliness is very important, otherwise there is no protection against illnesses. Use water for all occasions: when going to the toilet; and also before and after eating one should always wash hands, mouth and face. Water is the foundation of life. The more it is used, the more health will come.

Take salt before and after the meal, a small pinch is enough. It prevents many illnesses, as it activates digestion. That is part of the Divine Wisdom which has come to us through all the Prophets.

It is *sunna* not to sleep on the stomach. Best is to sleep on the right side or on your back, either facing the *qibla*, or placing your head in that direction. Holy people, who have fully submitted themselves to the Lord, have full confidence, and sleep on their backs. Never let babies or children sleep on their stomach. (see:COT-DEATH)

For your teeth you should use a *miswak*. Also rinse your mouth as much as possible with water and use a toothpowder made out of salt and ashes. For teeth it is also much better to use natural substances instead of chemical toothpaste.

Mankind must learn to come and declare their humbleness and their servanthood towards the Lord of Heavens. As long as they are not doing that, they will be punished and nothing will give them any treatment or health. The whole world can be filled with doctors and medicines and specialists, and still it will be impossible to give mankind any health or peace or satisfaction and to take away their sufferings. Without serving Him by obeying Him, that will be impossible. This must be well-known.

WHO PROFITS FROM ILLNESSES?

Big corporations do not want people to be healthy, because thousands of factories work to produce medicines. Only a small bottle of medicine costs a lot of money. There is so much trade from medicine. You cannot find a family which doesn't use medicine. Every family does! They use it for their children, adults, men, women, sick-ones or healthy-ones. They do not even leave the healthy-ones alone! They say to them that they have to take this and that as a check-up, or to prevent illnesses that could come. Everyone is being cheated to use tablets, or injections, or syrups. The goal is to make everyone a customer of the medicine factories, huge factories. People think that they cannot live without medicine. Once the idea has been established that life without medicine is not possible, people are even grateful for all the medicines. Sometimes there is no more medicine in our countries, so people are sent to Europe to get more tablets. Very often the medicine brought into the Third World is outdated, but they do not mind.

When people use herbs and everything which belongs to wild nature and hasn't been changed, they will find the best medicine. But it is now in fashion to use so many artificial medicines even though everything which has been made artificially harms the body. The worst is antibiotics. It fights the body, every cell is harmed by it. The doctors know, but patients have no patience and that is why doctors are obliged to give their patients such quick solutions.

So to have health it is important to use that which is healthy. People now do not use their physical body in a good way, but in the worst. So even the bodies of the young start to finish when they are 25 years old, because they are not using spiritual power to uphold their physical body. They are wasting their physical powers without thinking. That is why many are finished when they are only 25 years old. The power of the physical bodies of prophets and holy people never get weaker. Even if they are 100 years or more, it must be the same, because the spiritual power supports them.

In London there are milk-men. Their cars work with batteries, because they only go a few steps and then they stop. If they were using ordinary cars, the engine would burn out quickly. That is why they are using batteries. Those cars cannot be used on the motor way. And those who do not use their spiritual power are like that. Their bodies have only been trained to work with batteries. The power of the physical body will get weaker and weaker and weaker. So to use a battery for even 25 years is too much. But those who use spiritual power have atomic power.

There are aircraft that work with atomic power that can go around the world for 10 years or more. Spiritual power is even more than that. It enables people to live and be strong without problems until the end of their life. Spiritual power is the same in the end as in the beginning. It will never change. But people do not understand. They say, "No!" to all of this and then, when their battery has finished, they come to me and say, "Oh Sheik, I have no power..." I tell them, "You have burned your energy, it is finished! What can I do for you?"

CONDITIONS FOR THE SUCCESSFUL USE OF THIS BOOKLET

1. The acceptance of One Creator
2. No drinking of alcohol
3. No smoking of tobacco
4. To do or give a daily charity
5. When medicines are taken first thing in the morning, it is essential to wait one hour before eating or drinking anything else.

ALLERGIES

In summertime take a cold bath, in winter a hot. Drink a lot of *ayran* (a mixture of yoghurt, water and salt)

ANAEMA

Eat carrots cooked with raisins and sugar every morning and evening. Repeat for 40 days.

ANGINA

Rub vinegar on neck and head in the morning and in the evening. Keep warm: wear woollen socks and a woollen cap.

APPENDICITIS

Grind barley and boil with milk. Put it on the appendix area of the body once or twice while still hot. Leave it there the whole day and the whole night. Drink one cup of milk boiled with 5 ground cloves and mixed with honey, while still hot, in the morning, noon and evening.

ARTHRITIS

Boil sheep-trotters with plenty of water until it turns to jelly. Take some spoonfuls every morning before eating or drinking anything else. Repeat for 40 days.

ASTHMA

Take a handful of linseeds, grind them and boil with a *Turkish tea-glass* full of milk. Put the mixture on a cloth and cover the front from neck to belly and on the back from neck to waist. Cover with a woollen

garment and keep on overnight. Repeat 3, 5 or 7 nights.
and / or:
Take a radish, mash it and mix one spoonful of it with one spoon of honey and eat it. Repeat once in the morning and once in the evening for 15 days.

BABIES WHO HAVE DIFFICULTIES WITH SLEEPING
Restless babies have their restlessness transmitted from their parents' character. Give them aniseed tea and also a special *tawihs*.

BED WETTING
Take a big spoon of soapwort (saponaria officinalis) mixed with sugar before going to bed.

BIRTH POSITION
The best position, if you can do it, is squatting.

BLADDER / KIDNEY INFECTION
Take 5 kilos of cucumbers. Peel them. Take the skin and boil it with 3 bunches of parsley in a pot with twice as much water. When half of the water is boiled off, sieve it and put the juice into the fridge. Drink one *Turkish teaglass* full every morning, noon and evening until the infection is gone.

BLEEDING BETWEEN THE MENSES
Mix 1/2 tbl. spoon of melted butter and 1 tbl. spoon of honey and eat it first thing in the morning. Mostly this kind of bleeding comes as a punishment because

women hurt themselves before and during marriage in order to prevent having children. For this they use so many things. Be careful with this point if you don't want to be hurt, because the whole body-power of a woman lies in the womb. It is the most important part of their bodies and once they have hurt themselves there, doctors cannot do anything anymore. They are then like a broken dripping tap which cannot be mended.

BLOOD CLEANSING
Grind a handful of leaves from a sangalak-tree (Urdu: nima), mix with water, sieve and drink first thing in the morning. Repeat for 40 days.

BLOOD PRESSURE, HIGH
White cells in the old blood die all the time. The kidney cleans this. Sometimes when going into the veins the blood clots. So have your shoulders and head cupped 2 times a year, preferably in spring and autumn when it is not too hot or cold.

BLOOD PRESSURE, LOW
Eat a lot of salty things and meat with garlic and onions. Also 21 raisins with seeds first thing in the morning before eating or drinking anything else. Repeat for 40 days.

BLOOD TRANSFUSION

Instead of doing a blood transfusion clean your blood by drinking a soup of bonemarrow with black pepper, ginger, cinnamon and cloves.

BLOOD LOSS

Patience! Your body produces new blood by itself. Within 40 days the lost blood will be reproduced. Drink the same soup as in 'Blood transfusion' and also sheep milk with honey.

BRAIN CONCUSSION

1. Don't move and don't touch it!
2. Eat 21 raisins with seeds every morning.
3. Drink milk with honey, cold or warm, every morning, noon and evening.
4. Never allow an operation to be done.

BREASTFEEDING MOTHERS, LACK OF MILK

Wash some chick-peas, soak them overnight and in the morning drink the water in which they were soaked. Repeat daily until the milk becomes better.
It is also good to eat a lot of bananas.

BRONCHITIS

Dry the leaves of ribwort or coltsfoot (plantago lanceo) and its flowers. Then burn them and inhale with steaming water.

BULIMIA

In the days of the Romans it was a common practice for people to eat, then to use something to vomit, so that they could continue the pleasure of eating. Nowadays this phenomena is appearing in people as an illness.

Europeans do not eat in a normal way. For example: in the evening they go to a restaurant and they sit at least for 3 hours and more. They eat and drink and eat and drink for so many hours. They are only eating out of enjoyment, not out of necessity. The illness comes to them to make them come back to a normal life. They should eat when they need. If they do not need it, they shouldn't eat. People who suffer of bulemia should first stop to eat different kinds of food. They should not be mixing while they are eating. Their stomach does not accept mixed foods. They should eat only twice a day and drink barley water to prevent the vomiting. As long as they eat out of enjoyment the illness will never leave them. They should also never eat until they are full, but leave 1/3 empty. Within 40 days the illness will leave them. They should also try not to eat artificial hormones , but instead come back to simple foods: rice, wheat, barley, potatoes, vegetables... and all of it without hormones. Spices are all right, they prevent vomiting, especially thyme. Best is to take one tablespoon of thyme with salt every morning, chew it and afterwards drink a bit of water. Also drink hot drinks, don't drink alcohol or any fizzy artificial drinks. With every meal eat salad with salt, vinegar, olive oil and onions.

BURNS

Put cold water and then olive oil on the burn.

CAESARIAN

I don't believe that there are babies who don't come out. The only problem is that we are impatient. The One Who has planted the foetus in the womb of the mother must also bring it out. But we are not patient people.

Another reason why a lot of caesareans are done, is that people pay much more for a caesarean than for a normal birth. I don't believe that doctors do it for the best of the mothers. I don't believe that they are doing a good and a right thing.

Just last week I was saying, concerning my own daughter-in-law, "Don't do it, let her deliver the baby!" The gynaecologist said, "Everything is normal. But it is the first baby, so maybe the labour pains will last until tonight. Go to your home to rest and come back in the afternoon!" The mistake was, that Istanbul is too big a city to just go and come like that, so in the afternoon when the pain increased, she had to be taken to another hospital which was nearer. In the private ward two other gynaecologists had a look at her and said, "Oh, this is too much pain for her, her hands are already blue, which means it is dangerous. And the baby is upside down. The feet are at the bottom. What can we do?" The doctor in charge answered that a caesarean would be the only solution. Then, even though my daughter-in-law shouted that she did not want it, they did it.

The first doctor, who she had visited in the morning, said afterwards that everything had been all right and normal, also that the head had been lying like it should. He was the one who had been examining her all those months of pregnancy, so he should know. So I don't believe in doctors when it comes to deciding when to make a caesarean. They take money and cut.

CANCER
Every morning before eating or drinking anything else: drink 1/2 *Turkish tea-glass* full of freshly squeezed onion juice. Repeat for 40 days!

CHILDREN WHO DO NOT GROW
Pay *sadaqa*! Give them bone-marrow soup to eat and sheep's milk to drink.

CHOLERA
Don't eat or drink anything! Take Epsom-salt to clean yourself inside. Then drink a small cup of kerosene in the morning. No food during one day and if possible also no drink. If absolutely necessary, then drink the water of boiled unwashed rice.

CHOLESTEROL
The main reason for excess cholesterol is drinking wine. Wine collects the cholesterol in the blood like a magnet pulls iron together. Do not drink alcohol! With every meal eat a salad with onion and vinegar.
and / or: Boil a handful of leaves from a *loquat tree (Turkish: yeni dunya)* and drink several times a day.

COMPULSIVE WASHING

A full body wash is enough two times a day. If anyone needs more than that, then put your arms up to your elbows into a dustbin. Then cover face and head with the dirt of the dustbin. Leave it on the body for 10 minutes, then have a wash.

CONSTIPATION

Boil 3-5 figs in water. Drink the water and eat the figs before going to sleep.

CONTRACEPTION

The problem of mankind nowadays is that they do not believe. That is the root of nearly all their problems. These problems bring sufferings which make people unhappy and take away their peace and satisfaction. The problem of children is one of the biggest and it gives mankind a lot of suffering. Some people wish to have children and they can't. Others, like most young people, don't want any, neither before nor after the wedding. Illegal relationships are spreading all over the world and are destroying men and women physically and morally. Before marriage they are using contraception so that they will not have a baby as a result of their relationship. So they take a lot of poison to prevent getting pregnant. With this they are destroying themselves. Then, when they start a legal relationship after the illegal one, no children will be granted to them.

When Allah Almighty does grant a child, people often say, "One is enough!" or "Two are enough!" or

"Three are enough!" They don't want more than that, so they start taking contraception again. So what does Islam say to that?

First of all: Islam does not allow any illegal relationships. Then, there is only permission to use contraception under very special conditions. If it is clear that there would be danger to the life of the mother or the baby, or if the parents have an illness which could be inherited by the child, or by coming generations, then contraception is allowed.

But nowadays the reasons for contraception are purely personal. For example, women are afraid of getting children because motherhood does not fit into the situation in which most young girls find themselves nowadays. Once a woman is married, she wants to keep her figure and look like she did before she was married. Usually motherhood changes the figure. The way they want to look is usually the main reason for not wanting children.

The second reason is the financial one which forces most people not to want to have children. Most people don't believe that Allah Almighty has secured the provision for everyone and that their work and fate has been predestined. Most people are atheists and materialists who will never accept that Allah has created the children and that He will look after them. There is no reason to be worried. Just like we are living, Allah will let them live and will create suitable conditions for them in which to live. Their future is not like ours. The conditions for living are being changed every day, all the time. But unbelievers think that the same conditions will stay, and that is why they try to prevent children from being born. They kill them and this is a great sin.

The third reason is that women are not in the homes anymore. Cruel men force them to not only do the work in the house, but outside the house too. I have never seen such cruelty as in the 20th century, especially coming from men. Men also work outside, then they come home, sit down and relax. At the same time, women come home from work, and have to continue to work at home. At the age of 30 they already start to age.

And the silly women don't notice that the silly men are fooling them by telling them that men and women are equal and that they can be police-women, lawyers, doctors etc. The women just say, "yes" to all of that.

Then when these women have children, they don't even know their mothers properly, because except for a few hours, they are put in nurseries. They never experience the loving care and love of their mother, who by then is saying, "We need peace, two children are enough." Usually even one is enough for them.

Physically women who are working outside are made so weak that they do not feel encouraged to have more children. Islam takes the side of women when it says, "No work for women outside the house."

When I am given power, I will stop women from working outside their house. I will give them a salary for staying at home which will be higher than the one earned by the men working outside. Like that they will be happier inside than outside.

In Europe I see women who leave their houses in the morning darkness to catch a train or a bus, or who take a car to get to work. What is this cruelty good for? The whole responsibility is on the shoulders of men, but today most of them are representatives of the devil and they do not believe. I will punish those who let their women work outside. Also those who don't spend at least three hours a day with their children and wife.

In our days all conditions of communal life are based on cruelty and the women are forced to work. We have to change everything from A to Z and turn cruelty into justice and give women their rights. I am for all women staying at home without any exception. It does not mean that they should not be researching intellectually or develop whatever skills they have. They can do that, but without the pressure of having to earn money with it. Spiritually they have exactly the same duties as men, and the *hadith* to search for knowledge where ever you can, even if it means going to China, applies in the same way to women as to men.

COT DEATH

Cot deaths are results of *jinn* playing with the baby. So take all precautions:
1. Babies should, like grown-ups, never sleep on their stomachs. It should be either on the back or on the right side. Ideal is to have the head lying in the direction of the *qibla*, or to be facing the *qibla* when lying on the right side.
2. Let your baby wear the *tawihs* at all times.

3. Put a pillow or a cloth close to the baby with the colour red or purple, because these colours put *jinn* in a friendly mood.

4. Don't upset the *jinn* by doing housework after sunset. Especially work with water like mopping or laundry. *Jinn* are made of fire and any connection with water, especially after sunset when their day begins, upsets them. If it is necessary, then be very sure to invoke every action with a loud, *"Bismillah!"*

COUGH / BRONCHITIS

Before going to sleep at night:

1. Heat 3 tbl. spoons of olive oil.
2. Drench a big piece of cotton-wool with the hot olive oil.
3. Wrap it up in newspaper.
4. Put it on the chest while still hot.
5. Cover with a woollen sweater and leave until morning. Repeat for 10 nights. Also drink on cup of water and honey boiled with cloves, cinnamon, black pepper and ginger four times a day.

and / or:

Boil one big spoon of cornflour with a cup of milk. Add sugar and honey and drink hot before sleeping. Cover your head preferably with wool.

and / or:

Put *halva* paper (the paper in which *halva*, a Turkish sweet, is wrapped in) on your chest and on your back, cover with a woollen garment and leave overnight.

CRAMPS OF BABIES

In the old days it was a tradition that a prayer was said into the ears of a new-born baby. That was a tradition in all religions which has now been lost. To prevent cramps, and many other disturbances, do the following: call the *azahn*, the call for prayer, into the right ear and the *iqamat*, the smaller call for prayer, into the left ear. Also always give *sadaqa* for every birth. Keep the Holy Book above the sleeping place of the baby, use a red or purple coloured cover over their head as a protection against the *jinn* and use a *tawihs* at all times. If cramps should still occur, then give extra *sadaqa* and make a massage with olive oil.

CROSS EYE

Crush 3 cloves of garlic and mix with a spoon of honey. Eat every morning before eating or drinking anything else. Repeat for 40 days. If not gone, then repeat for another 40 days.

CROWNS

Don't have them made, because many infections can start underneath. Fillings are all right, also false teeth.

CURETTAGE

Anything taken away from the body, however small, makes the body abnormal and will give it trouble and pain and cause it to be incomplete. Curettage is the worst. Permission to do such a thing can only be given if a baby dies in the womb and they are obliged to remove it. If not, women who do that will be punished until the end of their lives. They are hurting their organ, and especially if the foetus is more than 4 months old, which means that it is also living in a spiritual sense, it is so dangerous to take away, and so cruel. It is like murdering it. Don't ever give permission to do such a thing.

In other cases when doctors advise to make a curettage the reason is that the organ has not been used in a good way. Every enjoyment has been made, and that which is prohibited, must be punished. Only if it happened before coming to Islam and before knowing that it is prohibited, then it is s different case. Then it is forgiven by Allah Almighty and the punishment is taken away. After someone has come to Islam, every *haram* action the person does will be punished and will bring trouble.

DANCER'S BONE

Mostly a problem of women. Don't use tight shoes. Your toes must be able to rest and to move. For treatment make a tight bandage around the toes, still enabling them to move. As long as you have the feeling that it is continuing to grow, keep making a bandage in this way. In general shoes must be comfortable to avoid illnesses of the feet.

DANDRUFF

Put olive oil and a little vinegar on the hair and massage the hair-roots with it. Leave it on the hair for one hour before washing it off.

DEAFNESS DUE TO DIRT IN THE EARS

Put hot olive oil into a syringe and drop 3 drops into each ear. After 2 minutes clean with cotton-wool.

DEPRESSION

Visit hospitals, mental-houses, prisons and old people's homes regularly and your own depressions will disappear quickly. Nowadays many young people get depressed because they are forced to make an education in which they have to learn theoretical subjects for long years which they afterwards never have to use. At the end of this uninspiring time they do not even get a job. To avoid this I suggest young people to learn skills like carpentry, which is very useful and will also give them a job at the end of their training.

DIABETES

Drink tea made of goose-grass (gallium aparine).
and / or:
Eat a lemon with the skin during one day. Repeat for 40 days.

DIARRHOEA

Take one big spoon of finely ground coffee and mix it with lemon-juice. Once swallowed it may be followed by a glass of water. After this no drinking or eating for several hours.

DISKS, WORN OUT

People should get used to eating the jelly which comes from cooking the trotters or the head of a sheep or cow. This jelly binds the bones together. People who eat this regularly provide their bodies with a storeroom of this. Every time the body needs it as a renovation, it will make use of it. It is like filling up the car with oil once the oil has been used. People who have a tendency of having problems with their disks should eat this jelly regularly every day, others every week.

DOG BITE

Put kerosene quickly on the would.

DRUG ABUSE

(like alcohol, tobacco, heroin, cocaine...)
The condition is that the drug abuser wants to stop and uses will power to do so. Take a bottle of water. Recite the first *sura* of the Holy Quran, *al Fatiha*, 40 times. After each *Fatiha* blow into the bottle of water. Every time when you feel an urge to use a drug, take a sip of the water instead.

EAR-ACHE

Take 1/4 teaspoon of black seeds (nigella sativa) and roast them and grind them. Add olive oil, heat it and put 7 drops with a syringe into the ear every morning and evening until better.

EPYEMA

Put a piece of tomato on the infection and tie a cloth around it overnight.

EPILEPSY

There are 2 main groups of epileptics:

1. Those possessed by *jinn*: if the attack is caused by *jinn* it is useful to put a piece of iron on the back of the neck until the attack is over. Any iron will do: knife, spoon... Always wear a *tawihs* covered in leather. Any *sura* or verse from the Holy Quran should be recited over them.

2. Dysfunction of the brain: this is sometimes caused by babies falling on their heads and it can then happen that they bleed in the head. This blood clots and damages the rest of the brain. These patients should be shaved on top of their head and be cupped. Only the clotted blood should be taken, not the clean. Repeat 3 times. Then take cow-gall and put it on the same place. Mix butter and black seeds (nigella sativa) in a thick paste and put on top. Tie the head for 3 days changing the head-band every 24 hours and putting some new mixture on it. One treatment is enough, *insha'Allah*.

EYE-INFECTION

Boil black tea and put on the eyes with cotton-wool, being very careful not to rub them, so that the infection does not spread. The best thing to do is to leave it on the eyes for about 15 minutes before sleeping. Another version is to bathe the eye in tea, for example in an egg-cup.

FEAR

This is connected to your spiritual life.

1. If you are an unbeliever you must start to believe, because no-one will give you peace except Allah.

2. If you are a believer you have no reason to fear if you have never harmed anyone. If you have, or if you did a disliked action, you must stop it because the harm will come back like a boomerang to you. If you insist on being rebellious, your fear will stay.

3. Believers should take a shower or a bath or just do *wudu* and pray. Unbelievers should sit down, close their eyes and be quiet.

Allah Almighty does not allow us to be tired of serving Him. We should always strive to do that, not be too tired. The angels are never too tired, they are always making *zikr*. If you are praising the Lord it will support your soul and the soul supports the body. When the spiritual support stops death will come. When the soul leaves the body it will die, because nothing supports it anymore. That is when you die.

According to the amount of *zikr* you do, you will find peace, happiness and satisfaction in yourself. The more time you spend with spirituality in the form of prayers and servanthood, you will find a secret happiness within yourself.

People are looking everywhere in the outside world to find happiness. But that is impossible. Even if they are kings, lords or the richest person on earth, materialistic things will never give satisfaction. Only the praising of the Lord will give satisfaction and more feelings of security concerning the future.

The more *zikr* you make, the more you will feel that you are protected. The coming days will be very difficult, dangerous and fearful. People will ask for security more and more and will start running to places where they think that they can be secure.

My *Grandsheik* said that when a dangerous situation comes to you run quickly to make *wudu* or take a bath. That will calm your nerves. If that is not enough, then take your praying-carpet, sit down on it, stand up on it and start to pray. This place will be the safest for you. The praying-carpet and prayers are the biggest protection now and in eternity.

In the First World War *Grandsheik* was a volunteer in the army. He told us that when he was in the Dardanelles there was the fiercest fighting going on. So many armies wanted to pass through. *Grandsheik* was there right until the end. Thousands died. He told us, "One day I was praying *duha* while enemies were attacking and throwing bombs at us. The biggest bomb of all came and exploded, because it was near to the main quarters of the army. Thirty seven people were killed. Everything was covered with dust. The general said, "Oh, our Sheik has died, the bomb fell exactly on his praying-carpet."

After the dust had settled, the general could see *Grandsheik* and how he was still praying in the distance. Nothing had happened to him, so the general was surprised and said to him, "What happened?"

"Nothing happened," said *Grandsheik*, "nothing that hadn't been ordered by Allah. I was praying *duha* and I had no fear. I did not look to the right or to the left."

The general said, "This prayer has rescued you. I swear, that when I come out of this I will not fail to do any of my prayers. Oh, *Hoca Effendi*, I am not praying out of fear of Allah, because so many times I have neglected my prayers and Allah did not punish me in any way. But now I fear that punishment could come from you."

Grandsheik says that as long as you are on the praying-carpet nothing evil can come to you. The first and the last protection for mankind is the praising of the Lord. So many terrible and dangerous days will be coming now. What you have seen until now is nothing compared to what will come. The people of that time will walk by the cemeteries and say, "Oh, you there under the soil, you are lucky not to see these days. I also wish to be with you there underneath." Terrible days are ahead of us. Believe in God and pray. Take your praying-rug, sit down on it and pray and praise the Lord. There is no other protection than this now. No army in the world can give you protection.

The angels are glorifying the Lord. They never tire to do so, because the glorifying is their food. The power of one angel is more than the power of all mankind. It is a special power. Compared to spiritual power weapons do not mean a thing. These can be stopped in one moment. One single person can stop all nuclear weapons in one single night, in one hour, in one moment. We are not afraid of a nuclear war. It will not be the way they want it to be. The control is in the hands of one Holy Person who is controlling everything. This world is under Heavenly Control. People think that they are the ones who are controlling it, but they are not controlling anything. The real control is in the hands of the 5 *qutubs*.

Allah commands us and He loves it when we glorify Him. It gives you energy and peace, it gives you everything. Try to spend more time doing so. Say more "*La illaha illallah*", more *salawat* and more "Allah, Allah..."

Try to spend more of your time for spiritual energy. Every prayer and every *zikr* will give you more energy and more strength and more love for Allah. Real life comes from love. When there is no love, there is no life. The Holy Ones say, that those who have no love are like dead people. Love is life, light and that which makes us complete. The more we have of it, the more our life will be complete and full of pleasure.

The main target of our *tariqat* is to train people to make more *zikr* and to take more power and support. The time for the Last Day is coming closer. Hundreds of signs have appeared, and one of them is that people have stopped praising the Lord. That is why so much suffering is coming to them. Then they ask for drugs. The cure for all illnesses is the glorification of the Lord. The love for Allah will give peace now and forever.

FIRST AID
1. Tie the wounds so as to avoid blood-loss.

2. Keep warm

3. Give fresh lemon juice or *ayran* (sour milk) to drink.

FUNGUS ON THE FEET

Don't leave your feet wet and see to it that your toes don't touch each other. When you are sleeping put buds of cotton-wool soaked in vinegar between your toes.

GALLSTONES

Drink a *Turkish tea-glass* full of radish juice every evening and morning. Continue the treatment for 15-40 days.

GLANDS

The main cause is coldness, therefore keep warm at all times. When infected: take a lemon and cut off the top. Put three pea-sized pieces of welding stone into the lemon. Put the lemon into warm ashes overnight. Boil camomile flowers and put into the lemon, then tie this stuffed lemon onto the upper disk of the backbone. Leave it there for 3 nights. If necessary repeat after a few days.

GNASHING OF TEETH

Before going to bed take a carob, tie a string at both ends, place the carob between your teeth and put the sting around your neck so that the carob can't fall out. Use it for three nights.

GOUT

Boil sheep trotters and drink as a soup several times a day.

HAIR-LOSS

When washing your hair only use olive oil soap or laurel soap. After washing it, rub the scalp with olive oil. For women: when in public try to cover the head to avoid the evil-eye.

HAY-FEVER

Every morning and evening put 3 drops of olive oil into each nostril. Cover your head at all times!

HEADACHE

There are so many reasons for headaches. It is important to find out why the head is hurting. Sometimes another illness in the body causes it. If that is not the case, then the reason is the nervous system in the neck hurting.

1. Massage head and neck.
2. Put a piece of material drenched in vinegar around your head.
3. Mix henna, cloves, mustard-seeds, black-seeds and senna pods together. Grind all of this and mix with vinegar. Put the mixture on the head and leave it for 2 days.
4. Cover your head at all times.
5. Boil 15 big brown beans, drink the water and eat the beans.

PREVENTING A HEART ATTACK

A heart-attack is a punishment for using our bodies without taking any care. The most harmful thing for the veins is smoking. Your veins never forgive you for smoking, so:
1. Stop smoking!
2. Eat as many quinces as possible: marmalade, salad, tea of the buds...(prepared in any way you like).
3. Don't worry!

HEART PROBLEMS IN GENERAL

Put a medium sized onion in a tin with hot ashes and heat on fire until the onion is roasted. Eat first thing in the morning. Repeat for 40 days. This is also a healing method for cleaning up the body after many years of smoking.

HEART BURN

Take a pinch of salt first thing in the morning and then drink the juice of 2 *turunges* (wild oranges). If not available, then grapefruit juice.

HAEMORRHOIDS

Chew 10-12 juniper berries first thing in the morning before eating or drinking anything else. Then drink a glass of water. Repeat for 15 days. If you don't have any teeth, then crush the berries before taking.

HICCUPS

Drink water.

HERPES

Drink a glass of *turunge* juice (wild oranges) or grapefruit juice every morning for 10 days.

WEAK IMMUNE SYSTEM

Eat 21 raisins with seeds every morning and plenty of almonds.

INFERTILITY

see: sterility

INSOMNIA

Never sleep between noon and sunset. Don't drink coffee or tea after sunset. Any time after sunset go to sleep at once when you feel sleepy. Respect your sleepiness, don't fight it. After 40 days of taking these precautions your sleeping problem will be solved, *insha'Allah*.

ISCHIATITIS

Heat salt and make a 10 minutes massage. After that a 10 minutes massage with olive oil. Tie the upper part of the body tightly with wool. Do this once daily before sleeping.

KIDNEY-STONES

Take a whole thyme-plant with the roots. Remove the leaves and wash it. Put it into a boiling pot of water and then take it off the fire. Leave the plant inside for one day. On the second day drink one glass full in the morning, at noon and in the evening. Continue the treatment until the kidney feels at rest.

KNEE-PAIN

Massage either with mustard oil or kerosene mixed with olive oil into the knee for 15 minutes every night. Then cover it with pure wool and leave overnight. Repeat for 15 nights.

LIVER AND GALLSTONES

Take a raw egg complete with a shell. Wash it, put it in a cup filled with pure lemon juice and cover the cup. Leave it overnight. In the morning the hard shell will have dissolved. Take the egg with the remaining thin skin carefully out of the cup and use it elsewhere. Drink the mixture of lemon juice and dissolved eggshell one or two days in a row without eating anything else.

FARSIGHTEDNESS

Crush one big or three small cloves of garlic and mix with one teaspoon of honey. Eat every morning one hour before eating or drinking anything else. Repeat for 40 days.

LUMBAGO

Fill a towel with heated salt and give a massage up and down from the place of pain downwards in the direction of your legs.

MALARIA
Take a big spoon of fluid quinine every day and cover the head with a cloth drenched in vinegar.

MASSAGE
When giving body massage heat crystal salt first, wrap it into a piece of cloth and then give the massage with it.

MEASLES
Eat a big spoon of carob-syrup three times daily. If not available, then apple-syrup. It is best if this is the only food during the illness.

MENISCUS
Give a massage of the knee every morning and every evening with a mixture of olive oil and kerosene. Then cover it with unwashed wool. Repeat for 7 days.

MENSTRUATION CRAMPS
For all illnesses of the female organs use 1/2 tbl. spoon of melted butter and mix it with 1 tbl. spoon of honey. Eat it first thing in the morning and wait for 1 hour before taking anything else.

MORBUS CHRON / CHOLITIS ULCEROSA CHRON
1. Roast, crush and mix 20-25 acorns and mix with glass of honey. Take one tbl. spoon every morning before eating or drinking anything else.

2. 1/2 to 1 hour later: mix stinging nettles (cooked like spinach) with cooked wheat, white beans and corn. Add sugar or salt, as you like.

3. Take a big spoon of olive oil one hour before lunch. Don't eat any meat or butter for 7 days, only vegetarian oil, best is olive oil. It is better to eat only dry things.

MOSQUITO BITES

Put paraffin on those parts of the body which are not covered before you go to bed. Should you have the unhealthy habit of sleeping in the nude, then take a bath in paraffin before sleeping.

MOUTH INFECTION VIRUS

Roast 2 teaspoons of black-seeds (nigella sativa). Then crush them and leave them in the mouth for 10-15 minutes. Repeat many times a day.

MUSCULAR DYSTROPHY

1. Make bone-marrow out of sheep-trotters and eat a spoon of it every morning, noon and evening.
2. Eat as many raisins with seeds as possible.
3. Crush and roast black seeds (nigella sativa), mix with natural honey and take a spoonful every morning, noon and evening.
4. Pay sadaqa.

MUMPS

Eat a big spoon of carob syrup every morning, noon and evening. Rub the infected area several times daily with olive oil.

NAIL-BITING
Put fingertips into chilli.

NEURODEMITIS
1. Drink a tbl. spoon of non-refined olive oil every morning.
2. Take a bath every day. Afterwards rub your whole body first with lemon and then with olive oil. Continue treatment until the illness disappears.

NOSE BLEEDING
Take the hard skin of almonds, roast it in the oven and crush into fine powder. Sniff!

OPERATIONS
There is never permission for cancer, heart or head operations. In fact, if anyone asks me, I don't give permission for any operations at all, because operations make your life shorter instead of longer.

Once the following happened to a family in Lebanon: a woman had a cancer operation. One year later she died. The daughter also became ill and went to hospital. Her son went as quickly as he could to Damascus to meet *Grandsheik Abdullah Daghistani.* Grandsheik gave him the advice to take to his mother out of hospital as soon as possible. This he did, even though the nurses and the doctors were running after him trying to prevent it. Twenty years later she was still well. It is a question of how strong your belief is, and the limits of this are different for everyone. Great belief gives you great certainty and patience and accordingly blessings. A weak belief will get even weaker in times of tests and trouble and leave you with no patience.

OVERWEIGHT

Eat a salad with plenty of vinegar every morning before eating or drinking anything else. Eat a breakfast one hour later consisting of either carbohydrates or proteins. Don't mix! During the rest of the day eat whatever you want. Continue this diet for 40 days.

PAINFUL AND BLEEDING NIPPLES
See: STRETCH-MARKS

PARALYSIS

1. Pay *sadaqa*.
2. Give a 10-20 massage with olive oil morning, noon and evening.
3. Crush *black seeds (nigella sativa)* and boil with water. Then mix with honey and drink as tea in the morning, noon and evening.

PARKINSON'S DISEASE

Before matters come to this point, people must take better care of themselves. They use their bodies in such a cheap way and very often do not care how they eat, sleep or work. This illness is a sign for a burnt out engine. People who have it must be patient. Then melt 3gr. of pure amber over fire on a teaspoon. Then take it away from the fire. The amber will become solid again, taking the shape of the spoon. Every time when you drink tea, coffee or water, stir it 3-4 times with that spoon before drinking. The spoon should last up to 1-2 months. Continue with the same treatment until the illness goes away.

PARODONTOSE
Brush your gums several times a day with a *miswak* until it bleeds. Continue this treatment for 3 days.

PASSING WIND
Drink aniseed-tea every morning, noon and evening.

PELVIS PAIN
Heat olive oil and massage.

PIMPLES
Often a sign of maturity and the need to get married. Give a massage of 5 minutes with olive oil and leave overnight.
or / and: put a leech on each pimple and leave until sucked full. It will then fall off by itself.
and / or: rub mustard-oil onto the whole body 3 times a week, 3 times daily.

PREGNANCY & ULTRASOUND (SCAN)
When a woman is pregnant it is not even advisable for her to go to the doctor. No-one's hand should reach the foetus. It is so wrong and against the Divine Rules. When Allah Almighty begins to create and to complete the foetus, angels are working on it. They never want doctors to look at what is inside. They want it to be left

as a trust. So don't go! It is the biggest mistake you can do, to go for a check-up every month when you are pregnant.

In the old days when the pains of birth came a midwife was called who then said, "*Bismillahi rahmani rahim*. Oh, my Lord, let your servant come!" That was all. I am against every form of control which the doctors are doing. Ultra-sound is a most dangerous thing to do for the foetus. It is unacceptable to disturb it in such a way. You never know which harm the radiation has caused to the child; if it goes through the eyes it can make them blind, through the ears make them deaf, through the mouth make them dumb...

Altogether ultra-sound is useless, even for cancer. The doctors do not know how to find a medicine to cure cancer, so they use ultra-sound. It is only good for them to earn more money. It is not a cure. That is why I am against the scan in general.

PROBLEMS OF MENOPAUSE
This comes from the nervous system so eat 21 raisins with seeds first thing in the morning.

PROLAPSED INTER VERTEBRAL DISCS
The patient should lie down on a hard surface on the stomach. Give a massage of the back with olive oil until some relief can be felt. The put a plaster on the place (one with holes which can breathe). On that put wool into the bend of the backbone so as to even it out and make it completely straight and to prevent any other movements. Then tie all of this tightly with a

bandage which should be at least 10-15 cm wide. During this procedure the patient should not move without assistance, someone else should do it for him. Keep this on for 40 days, or if necessary for 2 months. When taking a shower or a bath, take it off and put it on back afterwards.

PROSTATE

This is an illness which usually comes to elderly men as a result of their habit in keeping their urine too long. Every time when they have difficulties while urinating, they should prepare a container filled with some average warm water (40-50 C), and leave their organ inside while urinating.

PSORIASIS

Rub your skin two times daily with a lemon and then with olive oil.

PURIFICATION OF THE BODY AFTER TREATMENT WITH CORTISONE

Make a honey-syrup by mixing 3 spoons of natural honey into cold or hot water or milk. Use 3 times daily for 15 days.

REFLUX

This is when the acid of the stomach gets into your mouth. Drink the juice of wild oranges, *turunges*, in the morning. If that is not available, then grapefruit juice.

RHEUMATISM

Mix the excrement of bees with yogurth-whey until it is creamy. The rub onto rheumatic place and cover with pure wool.

RUNNING NOSE

Boil eucalyptus leaves in water and inhale several times a day.

SCAN

see: PREGNANCY AND ULTRASOUND

SCHIZOPHRENICS

They should always wear a *tawihs* and someone powerful should recite prayers and *suras* out of the Holy Quran over them for 40 days.

SCOLIOSIS

see: DISKS

SCORPION BITE

Put salt and saliva on the bite.

SEA-SICKNESS

1. Don't eat!
2. Lie down.
3. Sniff an onion.

SHOCK

Drink hot milk.

SHORT-SIGHTEDNESS
Every morning before eating or drinking anything else, eat 3 crushed cloves of garlic mixed with a spoon of honey. Repeat for 40 days.

SINUSITIS
Heat up olive oil with hot chilli. Put some drops into each nostril on cotton wool and then go to sleep. It may burn, but should be used several nights in a row.

SKIN-CANCER
1. Rub with cotton wool drenched in vinegar until it turns red, particularly at night before going to bed. Leave overnight.
2. Try to go as little as possible into the sun. If it should be necessary, then cover your skin completely. Take special care of also covering the face.

SLEEPWALKING
Tie hands and feet and shut windows and doors. Sleepwalking is caused by *jinn*, who want to take you for a walk.

SMOKER'S LEG
1. Every morning before eating or drinking anything else, drink a full cup of onion juice. Repeat until it feels better.
2. Mix olive oil and paraffin and give that part of the leg a strong massage for 15 minutes.
3. Eat a salad consisting of apple or orange with vinegar and oil every morning.

SNAKE BITE

Suck it out and tie something firmly around it. Then put lemon or vinegar on top, or put it in salty water until the pain goes.

SNORING

This is a problem of the structure of the nose. People who snore must test different positions of sleeping. For some it is better to sleep with, for others without a pillow. Snoring mostly occurs when people sleep on their back, so change your position! It usually helps a lot if people who snore go to bed with the intention of not snoring.

SORE THROAT / BEGINNING OF A COLD

Take some hot water, squeeze lemon juice inside and gargle every morning, noon and evening. Also drink this several times a day adding the lemon skin, honey and some crushed ginger.

SPRAINED ANKLE

Chop an onion and place the small pieces on the sprained area. Tie a piece of material around it firmly and leave it there for several hours. In severe cases repeat it many times until the swelling is gone.

STAMMERING

Take the eggshell of a swallow and use as a cup. Drink water in it several times a day saying, *"Bismillahi rahmani rahim."* every time.

STERILITY / INFERTILITY

Take 4 kg of dates and put them in a pot. Put twice as much water and let this boil until half of the water is gone. Wait until cooled down. Squeeze through piece of cloth and add to this juice 0.33 litres of carob juice. Keep in the fridge. Drink one *Turkish tea glass* full every morning and evening.

STIFFNESS IN THE FINGERS WHEN WAKING UP

This is a sign of weak nerves, so: eat 21 seedless raisins every morning before eating or drinking anything else. Before going to sleep rub your fingers with olive oil.

STOMACH ACHE

Drink peppermint tea. If hungry, then drink the water of boiled rice.

and / or: roast black seeds (nigella sativa) then mix with honey and eat.

and / or: take a big spoon of olive oil and drink.

and / or: grind 4 cloves into hot milk and drink with honey or sugar.

STRETCH-MARKS

Mix 1/3 glycerine, 1/3 lemon and 1/3 eau de cologne and massage into these places. This is also a good preventive when pregnant.

SUNBURN

Never stay directly in the sun. Rub your body with olive oil.

SUNSTROKE

Wash head and body with cold water.

TAPE WORM (INTESTINES)

Drink one cup of clear paraffin once a month until the worm comes out. It is important to see that the worm's head is out too, otherwise it regenerates itself.

TEARS, LACK OF, DRY EYES

Drink a tea made of elderberry syrup.

TENSIONS

a) If caused by a lot of physical work then give a massage to the nervous system.
b) If caused by inner reasons, nervousness, then make a lot of *zikr* and *salawat*.

TOOTHACHE

Heat vinegar with salt and gargle on the painful side.
or / and: put some crushed garlic into the hole.
or / and: chew up some clove and put it into the hole.

TORN MUSCLE

Move the joint as little as possible for 4 days. Give a strong massage with olive oil 3 times a day, each massage for 10-15 minutes. Wrap the joint with an elastic bandage.

TREMBLING BECAUSE OF OLD AGE

Melt some amber on a spoon and whenever something is drunk, whether cold or hot, stir the drink with the spoon of amber.

TUBERCULOSIS

Most sanatoriums for patients with this illness are in the pine woods, because the smell of pine trees give the ill power. Use the resin of the pine trees. Take some of it, boil it in water and drink the water 3 times daily. Use the same water as long as it has the bitter taste. When that is gone, then make a new mixture. Continue this treatment for 2 or 3 or up to 6 months, until it feels better. It renews the lungs and gives strength and health.

TUMOURS

To make an operation is never a treatment. Tumours grow in the body for a reason. Try to understand which kind of poison your body is trying to get rid of in this way. Something else can take it away, like onion juice. So: every morning before you eat or drink anything else drink the juice of one onion. After that do not eat or drink anything for 1 hour. Within 40 days your tumour should be cleaned away, *insha'Allah*.

ULCER

1. Take one spoon of *tahin*, sesame-cream, in the morning and in the evening.

2. Roast 21 acorns, grind them and mix with honey. Eat one spoonful in the morning and one before sleeping.

ULTRASOUND (SCAN)
see: PREGNANCY & ULTRASOUND

VACCINATIONS FOR INFANTS

These did not exist in the old days. The only vaccination I would suggest, is against chickenpox. Generally for every birth of a new child *sadaqa* should be paid, or if you slaughter a sheep it should be shared with others. If you are a believer, it is enough to give *sadaqa*, your child does not need vaccinations. When you are doing this say, "Oh my Lord, instead of giving the vaccination I am giving so and so much *sadaqa*, please accept it from me." This you repeat for every vaccination. Even if you do give the baby a vaccination you should give *sadaqa* as a protection, because with every vaccination you bring a poison into the body.

VERICOSE VEINS

Don't cut them, don't have an operation done. Give them a strong massage with olive oil and the surrounding area for 10-15 minutes. Repeat this every night for 40 nights. Pay *sadaqa*.

VAGINAL PARASITE

Mix one tbl. spoon of honey with 1/2 tbl. spoon of melted butter. Eat while still hot every morning before drinking or eating anything else. Repeat for 40 days.

WATER IN THE LEGS
Put a leech on the outer and inner ankle and leave them there until they fall off by themselves.

WARTS
Have someone spiritually powerful recite on them and pay *sadaqa*.

WEAK MEMORY
Eat 21 raisins with seed every morning and say, *"Bismillahi rahmani rahim"* with each one.

WISDOM TEETH
Have patience!

WOUND TREATMENT
Kerosene stops the bleeding and kills the bacteria. Always clean a wound with kerosene before tying it up.

YELLOW FEVER
1. Squeeze lemons and mix the juice with honey. Drink every morning, noon and evening as much as possible.
2. Pay *sadaqa*.
3. Eat rice with lemon.
4. Cover head and belly with cloths drenched in vinegar.

GLOSSARY OF TERMS

ayran: a yogurth type of sour milk which is often drunk in Mediterranean countries with water and salt.

azahn: the call to prayer.

bismillah: transliterated Arabic for "in the name of Allah"

bismillahi rahmani rahim: transliterated Arabic:"in the Name of Allah, most merciful, most compassionate"

duha: a voluntary prayer performed in mid-morning.

al Fatiha: the opening chapter of the Holy Quran.

Grandsheik Abdullah Daghistani: Sheik Nazim's Sheik, the 39th Sheik in the Golden Chain of the Naqshbandi Tariqat.

hadith: traditions and sayings of Muhammad* which have been precisely recorded and the chain of reporters can be traced to the origin.

halva: a Turkish sweet.

haram: that which is forbidden according to the Divine Rules.

Hoca Effendi: a respectful title for a leader in prayer.

insha'Allah: transcribed Arabic for "If Allah wills."

iqamat: the second call to prayer which announces that the prayer is just about to begin.

jinn: beings made of smokeless fire who inhabit the earth with us. They are like humans in the sense that they can be good or evil. They have responsibility with what they do because, like us, they have also been given will-power. The Holy Quran is addressing them too and they will be present on the Day of Judgement. Because they are made of a different material than we are, but we live on the same planet, it is important to know how to influence them, and not to annoy them unnecessarily. Their influence on us can be noticed in the energy surrounding us. If we are not in unity with the Creator, and we do not comply to His Rules, then they will enforce the feeling of fear. But if we are in unity, the presence of *jinn* can only enforce this reality and we will be even more in unity. Some people are more on the level of *jinn* and are more likely to get into contact with them. For them it is very vital to follow every means of protection: to say *bismillah* before any action, to have *wudu* at all times and to be careful not to cut hair or nails after sunset. When you cut them, always either burn or bury it into soil, a flower pot will do. Otherwise you invite the *jinn* to use it to put spells on you. (also see: COT-DEATH)

kufr: covering up the truth, not believing in the truth, falsehood.

la illaha illallah: transcribed Arabic for: no, there is no Allah but Allah.

loquat fruit: in Turkish, 'yeni dunya'. A yellow plum-sized fruit with two big pits.

miswag: a 6-10 inch piece of wood, often a twig of the araq tree or liquorice-root which is used to clean teeth.

qadr: predestined fate. The belief that everything has been planned by Allah.

qibla: the direction of prayer, the Kaaba in Mecca.

qutub: the spiritual pole, the axis of the world, the Man of Time.

sadaqa: charity. This can be in form of a donation or a good deed.

salawat: the plural of Arabic 'salat', prayer. In this case special prayers for the Prophet Muhammad*, asking for his support and protection.

sunna: The way and life of Muhammad*. People who follow the *sunna* try to copy the habits of Muhammad*. They are convinced that he was a living example of someone following the Divine Rules completely and so pleasing Allah and reaching to His Presence.

tahin: sesame-cream

tariqat: the way. Sufis are the mystics in Islam. They were originally divided up into 42 *tariqats*, ways to Heaven. These are practises which are taught by the leaders of the *tariqats*, the Sheiks, of how to reach to Heaven. It is important that these *tariqats* have a continuous line of succession leading back to the Prophet Muhammad*. In the case of the Naqshbandia Tariqat, Sheik Nazim is the 40th Sheik in this chain. We believe him to be the last one in this line of succession. The *hadith* has foretold that at the end of time all *tariqats* will dissolve but one, and that one will unite all *tariqats* under Mehdi Alehi Salam.

tawihs: a blessed protection amulet. It is very important that you get it from an authorised Sheik, who you can trust.

Turkish tea-glass: 0.3 cup, 0.075 pint, 60 cl.

turunges: wild oranges. In Europe they can be found in Turkish or Greek shops.

wudu: ritual washing of hands, mouth, nostrils, face, forearms, head, ears and feet with water so as to be pure for prayer.

zikr: remembrance and invocation of Allah, typical for Sufis, who by repeating the various Names of Allah, aim to get closer and closer to His Presence.

THE GOLDEN CHAIN OF THE NAQSHBANDIA TARIQAT

1. Sayyidina Muhammad, salla-lahu'alayhi wa salam
2. Abu Bakr Siddiqi Khalifat-Rasuli-lah
3. Salman al Farsi
4. Qasim Bin Muhammad Bin Abu Bakr as Siddiq
5. Imam Abu Muhammad Ja'far as Sadiq Bin Imam Muhammad al Baqir
6. Sultan-ul 'Arifin Abu Yazid Tayfour Bin 'Isa Bin Surushan Al Bistami
7. Abu-l Hasan al Kharaqani
8. Abu 'Ali Ahmad Bin Muhammad al Farmadi ar Rudhabari
9. Khwaja Abu Yaqoub Yusuf al Hamadani
10. Abu-l 'Abbas, Sayyidina Khidr 'Alayhi-salam
11. Khwaja 'Ala'u-d Dawlah 'Abdu-l Khaliq Bin 'Abdul Jamil al Ghujdawani
12. Khwaja 'Arif ar Riwgarawi
13. Khwaja Mahmoud al Faghnawi
14. Khwaja 'Azizan 'Ali ar Ramitani
15. Khwaja Muhammad Baba as Sammasi
16. Khwaja Sayyid Amir al Kulali
17. Imamu-Tariqati Baha'd Din an Naqshbandi
18. Khwaja 'Ala'u-d Din Attar al Bukhari
19. Khwaja Ya'qoub al Charkhi
20. Hadrat Ishan Khwaja-i Ahrar 'Baydu-llah
21. Muhammad az Zahid al Bukhari
22. Darwish Muhammad
23. Maulana Ahmad Kil Amkanaki as Samarkandi
24. Muhammad al Baqi'bi-lah Berang as Simaqi
25. Ahmad al Farouqi Sirhindi Mujaddidu-l Alfi Thani
26. Muhammad Ma'soum Bin Ahmad al Farouqi Sirhindi
27. Sayfu-d Din'Arif
28. Sayyid Nour Muhammad al Bada'uni
29. Shamsu-d Din Habibu-lah Jan-i Janan
30. Abdu-lah ad Dihlawi
31. Shayk Khalid Diya'u-Din al Baghdadi
32. Shayk Isma'il
33. Khas Muhammad
34. Shayk Muhammad Effendi Yaraqhi
35. Sayyid Jamalu-din al Ghumuqi al Husayni
36. Abu Ahmad as Sughuri
37. Abu Ahmad al Madani
38. Sayyid Sharafu-din Daghistani
39. Sultanu-l Auliya Abdu-lah al Fa'izi ad Daghistani
40. Sheik Muhammad Nazim al Haqqani Naqshbandia